Nitric Oxide

A Beginner's 3-Step Quick Start Overview and Guide on its Applications for Health, With a Sample FAQ

copyright © 2024 Patrick Marshwell

All rights reserved No part of this book may be reproduced, or stored in a retrieval system, or transmitted in any form or by any means, electronic, mechanical, photocopying, recording, or otherwise, without express written permission of the publisher.

Disclaimer

By reading this disclaimer, you are accepting the terms of the disclaimer in full. If you disagree with this disclaimer, please do not read the guide.

All of the content within this guide is provided for informational and educational purposes only, and should not be accepted as independent medical or other professional advice. The author is not a doctor, physician, nurse, mental health provider, or registered nutritionist/dietician. Therefore, using and reading this guide does not establish any form of a physician-patient relationship.

Always consult with a physician or another qualified health provider with any issues or questions you might have regarding any sort of medical condition. Do not ever disregard any qualified professional medical advice or delay seeking that advice because of anything you have read in this guide. The information in this guide is not intended to be any sort of medical advice and should not be used in lieu of any medical advice by a licensed and qualified medical professional.

The information in this guide has been compiled from a variety of known sources. However, the author cannot attest to or guarantee the accuracy of each source and thus should not be held liable for any errors or omissions.

You acknowledge that the publisher of this guide will not be held liable for any loss or damage of any kind incurred as a result of this guide or the reliance on any information provided within this guide. You acknowledge and agree that you assume all risk and responsibility for any action you undertake in response to the information in this guide.

Using this guide does not guarantee any particular result (e.g., weight loss or a cure). By reading this guide, you acknowledge that there are no guarantees to any specific outcome or results you can expect.

All product names, diet plans, or names used in this guide are for identification purposes only and are the property of their respective owners. The use of these names does not imply endorsement. All other trademarks cited herein are the property of their respective owners.

Where applicable, this guide is not intended to be a substitute for the original work of this diet plan and is, at most, a supplement to the original work for this diet plan and never a direct substitute. This guide is a personal expression of the facts of that diet plan.

Where applicable, persons shown in the cover images are stock photography models and the publisher has obtained the rights to use the images through license agreements with third-party stock image companies.

Table of Contents

Introduction	8
All About Nitric Oxide	10
Nitric Oxide as a Signaling Molecule	10
Production and Function of Nitric Oxide in the Body	12
Role of Nitric Oxide in Various Physiological Processes	15
Regulation of Nitric Oxide Levels	19
Health Benefits of Nitric Oxide	22
Improve Cardiovascular Health	22
Enhance Exercise Performance and Recovery	23
Regulation of Blood Pressure	24
Boost Immune Function	25
Management of Erectile Dysfunction	27
Improved Cognitive Function	28
Other Potential Health Benefits	29
Getting Started with Nitric Oxide	32
Step 1: Understanding your health goals	32
Step 2: Consulting with a healthcare professional	33
Step 3: Implementing lifestyle changes	33
Getting Nitric Oxide Through Foods	36
Natural sources of Nitric Oxide	36
Incorporating nitric oxide-boosting foods into your diet	38
Nitric Oxide Supplements: Pros and Cons	42
Advantages of Nitric Oxide supplements	42
Potential risks and side effects of Nitric Oxide Supplements	43
Proper dosage and usage guidelines	44
Choosing a reputable brand	45
Who should not be taking Nitric Oxide Supplements?	45
Nitric Oxide-Boosting Meal Recipes	49
Beet and Carrot Roast with Rosemary Garlic Butter	50

Overnight Nitric Oxide Oats	51
Garlic and Leafy Greens Stir-fry	52
Citrus Fruit Salad	53
Watermelon and Pomegranate Smoothie	54
Beetroot and Orange Salad	55
Spinach and Garlic Stuffed Chicken	56
Dark Chocolate Avocado Mousse	57
Pomegranate and Walnut Salad	58
Watermelon, Mint, and Feta Salad	59
Spinach Berry Lemon Smoothie	60
Pomegranate Refreshing Smoothie	61
Mediterranean Summer Salad	62
Energy Boost Smoothie	66
Anti-Diabetic Smoothie	67
Detox Juice	68
Spinach and Kale Blend	69
Strawberries and Elderberry Puree	70
Low FODMAP Blueberry Smoothie	71
Blueberry Flax Smoothie	72
Conclusion	**73**
FAQ	**75**
References and Helpful Links	**77**

Introduction

People are often baffled by different health conditions and they often seek various ways to deal with them. Just as expected, most of them seek the help of medical professionals—which is just as it should be because they know best, most of the time. Then, there are those who seek answers via alternative ways, either by completely changing their surroundings, lifestyles, or diet.

Do you ever wish to find an alternative treatment or therapy that will aid your athletic performance and make muscle fatigue recovery faster? Or are you someone who's in search of diet and lifestyle changes that will enhance your cognitive function and boost your immune health? Do you know someone who has a cardiovascular disease?

There is a simple molecule in your body that plays an important role in achieving all of the conditions mentioned above. By enhancing the production of this molecule, you are on your way to a healthy you.

This molecule is called Nitric Oxide, a signaling molecule that is responsible for promoting blood flow and enhancing nutrient distribution throughout your body.

In this guide, we'll discuss the following in full detail:

- What is Nitric Oxide?
- Role, production, and function of Nitric Oxide
- The health benefits of Nitric Oxide
- How to get started with nitric oxide
- Diet and lifestyle changes to increase Nitric oxide in your body
- Incorporating Nitric Oxide-boosting foods into your diet
- Pros and cons of Nitric Oxide supplements
- Who should not be taking Nitric Oxide supplements?
- Nitrate-rich meal recipes

Keep reading to unlock your knowledge about this simple yet essential molecule.

All About Nitric Oxide

For starters, Nitric Oxide is a gas formed when the nitrogen oxidizes. It is toxic and colorless. In this chapter, we'll tackle the main functions of Nitric Oxide in our body.

Nitric Oxide as a Signaling Molecule

Signaling molecules are substances released by the cells to communicate with each other for the regulation and coordination of the body's physical activities. There are several signaling molecules that the cells release including hormones, neurotransmitters, and gasses like Nitric Oxide.

Nitric Oxide is a simple molecule that plays an important function in many physiological activities within our body. It is one of the signaling molecules but with different characteristics and functions making it unique compared to hormones and neurotransmitters.

First, unlike the other two signaling molecules hormones and neurotransmitters, Nitric Oxide is gaseous. It is a free radical at the chemical level, meaning, it has unpaired electrons that constantly seek reaction.

Secondly, while hormones are released by glands into the bloodstream and affect distant cells, neurotransmitters are released by neurons and primarily influence adjacent cells. In contrast, Nitric Oxide is not stored but synthesized on demand and acts in a paracrine manner, meaning it influences nearby cells.

Furthermore, Nitric Oxide is soluble in lipids, allowing it to easily pass through cell membranes without the need for specific transporters or receptors, unlike many other signaling molecules. Once produced, Nitric Oxide diffuses rapidly in all directions, influencing not only the cell in which it was produced but also neighboring cells.

Another key difference of Nitric Oxide is that through the process called nitrosylation, it directly affects proteins giving way to rapid and localized response. Hormones and neurotransmitters, on the other hand, require specific receptors where they can bind before they can make an impact on proteins.

These characteristics of Nitric Oxide allow it to serve as a versatile signaling molecule involved in several physiological processes. It plays a critical role in a variety of biological actions including neurotransmission, immune response, and regulation of cell death. Moreover, it is a major player in the cardiovascular system where it regulates blood pressure by relaxing the smooth muscle in blood vessel walls, leading to vasodilation.

Overall, Nitric Oxide is a simple yet important signaling molecule that is crucial for several body functions.

Production and Function of Nitric Oxide in the Body

Nitric Oxide (NO) is synthesized in the body through a complex process involving a group of enzymes known as nitric oxide synthases (NOS). There are three isoforms of NOS: endothelial NOS (eNOS), neuronal NOS (nNOS), and inducible NOS (iNOS). Each isoform has specific functions and is localized in different tissues and organs.

The production of Nitric Oxide begins with the conversion of the amino acid L-arginine into NO and L-citrulline, catalyzed by NOS. This enzymatic reaction requires several cofactors, including oxygen, nicotinamide adenine dinucleotide phosphate (NADPH), and various proteins. Importantly, NOS requires calcium and calmodulin for its activation, which provides tight regulation over NO production.

The endothelial isoform, eNOS, is primarily found in endothelial cells lining the blood vessels. It plays a crucial role in regulating vascular tone and blood flow. Under normal physiological conditions, eNOS produces small amounts of NO, which helps to maintain proper vascular function and prevent the formation of blood clots. Factors such as shear stress, which occurs during physical exercise, can stimulate eNOS activity and increase NO production.

The neuronal isoform, nNOS, is mainly present in neurons of the central and peripheral nervous systems. It participates in neurotransmission, playing a role in memory formation, learning, and the regulation of smooth muscle tone in the gastrointestinal tract. nNOS is activated by calcium influx into neurons and is involved in the release of NO as a neurotransmitter. This facilitates communication between neurons and contributes to various physiological processes.

In contrast, the inducible isoform, iNOS, is not constitutively expressed in most tissues under normal conditions. Instead, its expression is induced by inflammatory stimuli such as bacterial endotoxins, cytokines, and oxidative stress. iNOS produces large amounts of NO, which is required for the immune response against pathogens. While the acute release of NO by iNOS can be beneficial in fighting infections, excessive and prolonged NO production can cause tissue damage and contribute to inflammatory diseases.

The production of Nitric Oxide is influenced by various factors, including diet and exercise. Certain nutrients, such as L-arginine, the precursor of NO, can enhance NOS activity and increase NO production. Foods rich in L-arginine include nuts, seeds, legumes, and meat. Additionally, antioxidants like vitamins C and E can help to maintain the availability of NO by preventing its breakdown by reactive oxygen species.

Exercise also plays a significant role in modulating NO production. Physical activity increases blood flow and shear stress, leading to the activation of eNOS in the endothelial cells lining the blood vessels. This results in increased NO synthesis, promoting vasodilation and improving cardiovascular health. Regular exercise has been shown to enhance NOS activity, improve blood flow, and reduce the risk of cardiovascular diseases.

The localization and distribution of Nitric Oxide production vary in different tissues and organs. In addition to the endothelium, eNOS is found in other cell types, including platelets, smooth muscle cells, and cardiomyocytes. The neuronal isoform, nNOS, is present in neurons throughout the central and peripheral nervous systems. It is particularly abundant in regions involved in memory, learning, and motor control. iNOS, on the other hand, is primarily expressed in immune cells, such as macrophages and neutrophils, during inflammation.

In conclusion, Nitric Oxide is synthesized in the body through the action of nitric oxide synthase enzymes. These enzymes convert L-arginine into NO and L-citrulline, requiring various cofactors for their activity. The different isoforms of NOS, including eNOS, nNOS, and iNOS, are localized in specific tissues and have distinct functions. Factors such as diet and exercise can influence NO production. Understanding the production and function of Nitric Oxide in the body is essential for comprehending its role in physiological processes and its potential therapeutic applications.

Role of Nitric Oxide in Various Physiological Processes

In this section, we'll talk about how Nitric Oxide works inside our body, specifically its roles in various physiological processes.

Nitric Oxide's role in vasodilation and blood flow regulation

This function of Nitric Oxide is beneficial in maintaining cardiovascular health. Through the endothelial nitric oxide synthase (eNOS), Nitric Oxide is released by endothelial cells that are lining the blood vessels. The Nitric Oxide then acts as a signaling molecule that relaxes and widens the soft muscle surrounding the blood vessels resulting in an increased blood flow and enhanced oxygen distribution to tissues.

Prevention of hypertension and atherosclerosis

Hypertension or high blood pressure has been linked to the decrease of Nitric Oxide in the body. As previously discussed, Nitric Oxide plays an important function in vasodilation that aids in improving the blood flow. The absence of Nitric Oxide can result in vasoconstriction wherein the blood vessels are constricted leading to poor blood flow and high blood pressure. Similarly, Nitric Oxide also keeps the white blood cells from sticking to the endothelial cells or the cells lining the blood vessels. This process helps reduce the formation of atherosclerotic plaques that cause the thickening of arterial walls leading to high blood pressure. Thus, Nitric Oxide is essential in maintaining blood pressure.

Involvement of nitric oxide in immune response and defense mechanisms

Nitric Oxide is also beneficial to immune health. As a response to infections or inflammation, the white blood cells known as macrophages and neutrophils produce inducible Nitric Oxide or iNOS. These iNOS release high levels of Nitric Oxide that acts as an antimicrobial agent to stop the infection from spreading by inhibiting the growth and replication of pathogens. Nitric oxide also boosts the ability of these white blood cells to kill infections, enhancing the immune system.

Nitric Oxide's influence on neurotransmission, memory, and cognitive function

Nitric Oxide could also function as a neurotransmitter signaling molecule through the Neuronal nitric oxide synthase or nNOS that synthesizes the NO in neurons. As a signaling molecule, NO facilitates the communication and connections between the neurons enhancing the brain's cognitive functions including learning, memory formation, and motor control. Thus, NO is a vital signaling molecule that enhances cognitive functions and neurological health.

Nitric oxide's role in platelet aggregation and clotting processes

When the blood vessel is damaged, say at the time of injury, the platelets keep you from excessive bleeding. Platelets attach to the exposed collagen and form aggregates to create a clot. This blood clotting has pros and cons. It can stop excessive blood loss but if not regulated, platelet aggregates could obstruct the blood vessels known as thrombosis. This condition could lead to a heart attack if a thrombus forms in the coronary artery, the artery that supplies blood to the heart.

This is where Nitric Oxide comes in. Nitric Oxide prevents the adherence of platelet aggregates to the blood vessels and maintains blood flow. NO does this by acting as an enzyme that leads to the production of cyclic guanosine monophosphate (cGMP), a cyclic nucleotide that promotes muscle relaxation and inhibits platelet activation.

Impact of nitric oxide on inflammation and oxidative stress

Nitric Oxide's role in inflammation and oxidative stress is a complex one. For one, NO can act as an antioxidant that combats pathogens and inflammation. However, excessive

NO production can lead to tissue damage and chronic inflammation.

Inflammation is a body's response to infection or injury. When the tissues are injured or infected, the immune cells or white blood cells release inducible nitric oxide synthase or iNOS which also gives off a large amount of nitric oxide as a response against infection.

On the other hand, oxidative stress occurs when there is an excessive production of reactive oxygen species or ROS and the body's ability to combat its harmful impacts is insufficient. ROS are oxygen-free radicals that are highly reactive and are linked to contributing to the aging process and various diseases including cardiovascular disease.

Nitric oxide can help to counteract oxidative stress by acting as an antioxidant that neutralizes oxygen free radicals. However, it's important to note that this process could result in the production of reactive nitrogen species or RNS which is a potent oxidant known to damage lipids, proteins, and DNA cells.

This is how complex the role of NO in inflammation and oxidative stress is. It can either be harmful or helpful. Having this knowledge can lead to the right judgment in the treatment process of various diseases associated with inflammation and oxidative stress.

Potential implications of nitric oxide in metabolic processes and glucose homeostasis

Finally, Nitric Oxide has been linked to the regulation of blood sugar levels and metabolic disorders such as diabetes. Nitric oxide can enhance insulin sensitivity and promote glucose uptake in the skeletal muscle cells.

In conclusion, nitric oxide plays a multifaceted role in various physiological processes within the human body. From regulating vasodilation and blood flow to influencing immune response, neurotransmission, platelet function, inflammation, and oxidative stress, NO impacts diverse aspects of human health. The understanding of nitric oxide's functions opens up avenues for potential therapeutic applications and highlights its significance in maintaining overall well-being.

Regulation of Nitric Oxide Levels

Nitric oxide (NO) is a critical signaling molecule in the body, playing pivotal roles in various physiological processes such as vasodilation, neurotransmission, and immune responses. However, its levels need to be tightly regulated as an imbalance can lead to pathological conditions including cardiovascular diseases, neurodegenerative disorders, and chronic inflammation. Several factors influence the production and bioavailability of NO in the body and its breakdown.

The creation of NO is mainly overseen by a group of enzymes called nitric oxide synthases (NOS). These enzymes come in three different forms: inducible (iNOS), neuronal (nNOS), and endothelial (eNOS). Each isoform is regulated differently and is expressed in different cell types, contributing to the complexity of NO regulation. nNOS and eNOS are constitutively expressed and produce NO in response to physiological stimuli, while iNOS is induced during inflammatory responses and produces large amounts of NO. The activity of these enzymes is influenced by various factors, including the availability of substrates and cofactors, post-translational modifications, and interactions with other proteins.

Several molecules can modulate NO synthesis. For instance, the amino acid L-arginine is a substrate for NOS and its availability directly impacts NO production. Additionally, tetrahydrobiopterin (BH4), a cofactor for NOS, is crucial for enzymatic activity. A deficiency in BH4 can cause NOS to become "uncoupled," leading to reduced NO production and increased production of reactive oxygen species (ROS).

Once produced, NO is rapidly diffused and reacts with various biomolecules, limiting its lifespan. However, certain molecules can scavenge NO and prolong its bioavailability. For example, superoxide dismutase (SOD) catalyzes the dismutation of superoxide, a ROS that reacts with NO to form peroxynitrite, a potent oxidant. By reducing superoxide levels, SOD preserves NO bioavailability and prevents oxidative stress.

Furthermore, the breakdown of NO is also regulated. NO can be oxidized to nitrite and nitrate by oxyhemoglobin in red blood cells and by other heme-containing proteins. These reactions not only remove NO but also generate reservoirs of nitrite and nitrate that can be reduced back to NO under certain conditions, providing another layer of regulation.

Antioxidants also play a critical role in maintaining NO balance. As mentioned, NO can react with ROS to form reactive nitrogen species (RNS), which can cause cellular damage. Antioxidants can neutralize ROS and RNS, preventing their harmful effects. Moreover, some antioxidants, like ascorbic acid (vitamin C), can preserve NO bioavailability by reducing nitrite back to NO.

In conclusion, the regulation of NO levels in the body is a complex process involving multiple factors that influence its production, bioavailability, and breakdown. Understanding these regulatory mechanisms is crucial for developing therapeutic strategies targeting NO signaling in various diseases.

Health Benefits of Nitric Oxide

Now that we have a wider grasp of the role of Nitric Oxide in our body and how it works, let's dive into its benefits.

Improve Cardiovascular Health

It is known that cardiovascular diseases such as stroke and heart disease are the leading cause of death worldwide. Fortunately, there are several lifestyle changes that you could follow to avoid acquiring cardiovascular diseases. One of these is enhancing the production of Nitric Oxide in your body.

As discussed, Nitric Oxide aids in blood vessel dilation or causes the blood vessels in the body to widen. This enhances the blood flow and circulation throughout the body and is very beneficial in preventing high blood pressure.

This enhanced blood flow also aids in preventing plaques from building up inside the arteries. Plaque build-ups are the leading cause of stroke and heart disease.

Furthermore, Nitric Oxide also plays a crucial role during injury by regulating the blood clots. Blood clots, if unregulated, can block blood vessels which will lead to serious health problems.

Given all these roles of Nitric Oxide, it is worth noting that this signaling molecule is beneficial in preventing cardiovascular diseases.

Enhance Exercise Performance and Recovery

Nitric oxide (NO) is a vital molecule in the human body that plays a key role in various physiological processes, including blood flow regulation, immune response, and neurotransmission.

One of the primary benefits of NO is its ability to increase the delivery of nutrients and oxygen to muscles during exercise. This is made possible by Nitric Oxide's ability to enhance blood flow which equally improves the nutrient distribution throughout the body.

In addition to improving blood flow, NO has also been shown to improve muscle efficiency and endurance. This is due to NO's ability to stimulate the production of mitochondria, the energy-producing organelles within cells. By increasing the number of mitochondria, NO can improve the capacity of muscles to use oxygen and produce energy, leading to improved endurance and performance.

NO can also help to reduce exercise-induced fatigue, which is a common side effect of intense or prolonged workouts. This is because NO can increase the delivery of oxygen and nutrients to the muscles, reducing the buildup of metabolic waste products that can contribute to fatigue. Additionally, NO can help to improve muscle contractility, reducing the energy required for muscle contractions and further delaying the onset of fatigue.

Another benefit of NO is its ability to accelerate recovery after intense workouts. Exercise-induced muscle damage and inflammation can lead to soreness and reduced performance in subsequent workouts. However, NO supplementation has been shown to reduce inflammation and oxidative stress, promoting faster recovery times and reducing the risk of injury.

Overall, it is found that Nitric Oxide is beneficial to fitness enthusiasts in aiding throughout their physical activities.

Regulation of Blood Pressure

As mentioned above, Nitric Oxide is a key molecule in vasodilation, or the widening of blood vessels that regulates blood flow. This is beneficial in the regulation of blood pressure for those who have hypertension.

In addition to the vasodilation effect of NO, it is also found that it lowers systemic vascular resistance. Systemic vascular resistance is the resistance that blood encounters as it flows through the blood vessels. By lowering the systemic vascular resistance, the heart exerts less effort in pumping blood throughout the body.

Boost Immune Function

Nitric oxide (NO) plays a vital role in the functioning of the immune system. Here are five key points about NO and its impact on immune function:

Nitric Oxide's role as a signaling molecule in the immune system

NO is produced by a variety of immune cells, including macrophages, neutrophils, and dendritic cells. Once produced, NO acts as a signaling molecule that can influence the activity of other immune cells and regulate immune responses.

Activation of immune cells and defense mechanisms

NO can activate immune cells and stimulate a wide range of defense mechanisms, including phagocytosis (the process by which immune cells engulf and destroy pathogens), oxidative burst (the release of reactive oxygen species to kill pathogens), and cytokine production (the release of signaling molecules that coordinate immune responses).

Enhanced ability to fight off infections and pathogens

By promoting immune cell activation and defense mechanisms, NO can enhance the body's ability to fight off infections and pathogens. Studies have shown that NO can be effective against a wide range of pathogens, including viruses, bacteria, and fungi.

Potential benefits for individuals with weakened immune systems

Due to its ability to enhance immune function, NO may offer potential benefits for individuals with weakened immune systems, such as those with autoimmune diseases or HIV/AIDS. However, more research is needed to fully understand the potential benefits and risks of NO supplementation in these populations.

Considerations for supporting immune health through nitric oxide modulation

While NO can play an important role in immune function, excessive or prolonged NO production can have negative effects on immune cells and lead to chronic inflammation. As such, it is important to support immune health through balanced regulation of NO production and modulation. This can be achieved through lifestyle factors such as diet, exercise, and stress management, as well as targeted supplementation with NO precursors or modulators under the guidance of a healthcare professional.

Management of Erectile Dysfunction

Nitric oxide is a vital player in managing erectile dysfunction, serving as the primary vasoactive nonadrenergic and noncholinergic neurotransmitter that aids male organ erection. Its main role is to act as a vasodilator, relaxing the inner muscles of blood vessels, including those in the male organ, thereby widening them and increasing blood flow, which is crucial for achieving and maintaining an erection.

Research indicates nitric oxide's importance in facilitating erections by relaxing the vascular muscle supplying the male organ with blood. It is released by cells in the corpora cavernosa of the male organ, activating the necessary physiological mechanisms for an erection. When there's a decline in nitric oxide activity, often seen with certain risk factors or aging, it can lead to erectile dysfunction.

Supplements like L-citrulline, L-arginine, and French maritime pine bark extract, which boost nitric oxide levels in the body, can potentially improve erectile function. These supplements function by enhancing nitric oxide production, thereby facilitating the relaxation of the corpus cavernosum and boosting blood flow to produce erections.

However, it's noteworthy that while nitric oxide supplements can be beneficial, they should be used as part of a comprehensive treatment plan that may also include lifestyle modifications, other medications, and possibly psychological counseling. Always consult with a healthcare professional before starting any new supplement regimen, especially if you have underlying health conditions.

In summary, nitric oxide is integral to the physiological process of achieving an erection. Its role in increasing blood flow to the male organ makes it critical for sexual health. With aging and certain risk factors, nitric oxide activity may decline, potentially leading to erectile dysfunction. However, nitric oxide supplements, along with other treatments, can help manage this condition by improving the body's nitric oxide levels and enhancing erectile function.

Improved Cognitive Function

In addition to improving cardiovascular health, enhancing exercise performance, and boosting immune function, Nitric Oxide is also beneficial in improving the cognitive function of the brain.

By improving blood flow, Nitric Oxide equally enhances the oxygen distribution to the brain which is beneficial in providing the essential nutrients that the brain needs.

Furthermore, NO is a signaling molecule that plays a critical role in neurotransmission, the process by which neurons communicate with each other in the brain. By regulating neurotransmitter release and receptor activity, NO can influence a wide range of brain functions, including learning, memory, and mood.

Due to its role in neurotransmission and blood flow regulation, NO may offer potential benefits for memory, focus, and mental clarity. Studies have shown that NO-promoting substances can improve cognitive function in healthy individuals and those with cognitive impairment.

Lastly, NO has been shown to have neuroprotective effects, meaning that it can protect neurons from damage and degeneration. This has potential implications for neurodegenerative diseases such as Alzheimer's and Parkinson's, which are characterized by neuronal damage and death.

Ultimately, Nitric Oxide is a key factor in enhancing the cognitive function of the brain by enhancing neurotransmission, blood flow, oxygen, and nutrient distribution, and protecting neurons from damage and degeneration.

Other Potential Health Benefits

In addition to its well-known roles in immune function and cardiovascular health, NO also has potential applications in a variety of other areas of health and wellness. Here are five potential health benefits of nitric oxide:

Nitric oxide's role in wound healing and tissue repair: NO has been shown to play an important role in wound healing and tissue repair by promoting the growth of new blood vessels and enhancing the migration and activity of cells involved in tissue regeneration. This has potential implications for the treatment of chronic wounds and other injuries.

Potential benefits for individuals with diabetes or metabolic disorders: NO can improve insulin sensitivity and glucose uptake in cells, which may be beneficial for individuals with diabetes or other metabolic disorders. NO can also reduce oxidative stress and inflammation, which are factors that contribute to the development of these conditions.

Effects on erectile function and sexual health: NO is a key signaling molecule involved in the dilation of blood vessels, including those in the penis. By promoting blood flow to the genital region, NO can improve erectile function and sexual health in men. Additionally, NO has been shown to have potential applications in female sexual health, including improving lubrication and reducing pain during intercourse.

Role in gastrointestinal health and digestion: NO is involved in regulating the function of smooth muscle in the digestive tract, which can affect digestion and bowel movements. Emerging research suggests that NO may have potential applications in the treatment of conditions such as irritable bowel syndrome (IBS) and inflammatory bowel disease (IBD).

Emerging research and ongoing studies on nitric oxide's potential applications: In addition to the areas of health and wellness mentioned above, there is ongoing research on the potential applications of NO in a variety of other areas, including cancer treatment, bone health, and skin health.

It is important to note that while NO shows promise in these areas, more research is needed to fully understand its potential benefits and risks. Additionally, while NO can be beneficial in certain contexts, excessive or prolonged NO production can have negative effects on health, including contributing to oxidative stress and inflammation.

Getting Started with Nitric Oxide

After discovering the wonders that Nitric Oxide does to our body, are you now keen to get started on how to enhance the production of Nitric Oxide in your body? In this 3-step guide, let's dive deep into the things that you can start taking action on at this moment.

Step 1: Understanding your health goals

After understanding the roles and benefits of Nitric Oxide, the first step to getting started with it is to identify your health goals. Based on the health benefits mentioned above, what are you trying to achieve as far as Nitric Oxide can do? Are you an athlete doing robust physical activities daily and looking for ways to recover from fatigue or enhance your exercise performance? Are you someone with cardiovascular disease seeking natural alternatives to manage your condition? Do you want to improve your immunity and cognitive health?

Before jumping into the ways on how you could improve the Nitric Oxide production in your body, it is important that you do a self-introspection to motivate you in achieving your health goals. After all, you're doing this for your overall well-being.

Step 2: Consulting with a healthcare professional

Now that you have a clear vision of the health goals that you want to achieve with Nitric Oxide, it is best to discuss this with a healthcare professional. While this guide provides you with the necessary education you need about Nitric Oxide, it is important to note that this doesn't serve as a substitution for professional advice.

Your doctor is the best person who can guide you with your health goals. It is best that you discuss your goals, concerns, and health background with a healthcare professional for a tailored treatment suited for you. This is exactly true if your condition calls for Nitric Oxide supplements. In this case, your doctor can guide you on the right Nitric Oxide dosage to take.

Step 3: Implementing lifestyle changes

Regardless if your condition requires you to take Nitric Oxide supplements, your doctor will surely recommend these lifestyle changes to enhance the Nitric Oxide production in your body:

Exercise: Regular exercise is a powerful way to increase NO production in the body. Exercise promotes the release of certain hormones and growth factors that stimulate NO production, as well as increases blood flow and oxygenation, which can support NO synthesis. Studies have shown that both aerobic and resistance exercise can increase NO production, with benefits seen even after a single session.

Diet: Certain foods can help to increase NO production in the body. Foods that are high in nitrates, such as leafy greens, beets, and other veggies, can be converted to NO in the body. Foods that are high in antioxidants, such as berries, dark chocolate, and green tea, can also help to support NO synthesis by reducing oxidative stress.

Sunlight exposure: Exposure to sunlight can help to increase NO production in the body. Sunlight triggers the release of a molecule called urocanic acid in the skin, which can stimulate NO production. However, it is important to balance sunlight exposure with proper sun protection, as excessive sun exposure can increase the risk of skin damage and cancer.

Stress reduction: Chronic stress can suppress NO production in the body, so it is important to manage stress levels to support healthy NO levels. Techniques such as meditation, deep breathing, yoga, and mindfulness can all help to reduce stress and promote NO synthesis.

Sleep: Poor sleep quality and duration can also negatively impact NO production in the body, so it is important to prioritize adequate and quality sleep. Strive to get between 7 and 8 hours of slumber each night, and cultivate healthy sleep habits. These may include steering clear of screens before going to bed, maintaining a regular sleep routine, and establishing a cozy environment conducive to sleep.

Hydration: Adequate hydration is also necessary for healthy NO production. Drinking enough water can help to support blood flow and oxygenation, which are key factors in NO synthesis. Aim to drink at least 8 cups of water per day, and more if you are exercising or in a hot climate.

Smoking cessation: Smoking is a major contributor to oxidative stress and inflammation in the body, both of which can negatively impact NO production. Quitting smoking can help to reduce these risks and support healthy NO levels.

Overall, lifestyle changes such as exercise, diet, sunlight exposure, stress reduction, sleep, hydration, and smoking cessation can all help to support healthy NO levels in the body. By promoting NO production, these strategies have the potential to improve health outcomes across a variety of domains, including cardiovascular health, immune function, cognitive function, and more.

Getting Nitric Oxide Through Foods

While there are supplements and medication to increase your Nitric Oxide, there are heaps of foods that you can incorporate into your diet that will aid in increasing your Nitric Oxide.

Natural sources of Nitric Oxide

Although Nitric Oxide is not readily available in any foods, there are certain foods that contain nitrates which can be converted into Nitric Oxide once it enters your digestive system. Here are some of the natural nitrate sources:

Garlic: Garlic is a common spice for cooking and is known to be rich in amino acids that can be converted into Nitric Oxide in the body.

Spinach: This green leafy vegetable is not only an excellent source of iron but is also rich in nitrates that can increase the Nitric Oxide levels in the body.

Beets: This vibrantly red vegetable is not only delicious but is also rich in nutrients beneficial for your health. One of these nutrients is the nitrates necessary for Nitric Oxide production in the body.

Citrus fruits: Citrus fruits such as oranges, lemons, and grapefruits are known as sources of vitamin C but they are also excellent sources of flavonoids which aid in increasing the Nitric Oxide in your body.

Pomegranates: This fiber-rich fruit is also rich in nitrates and other compounds that help in Nitric Oxide production.

Leafy greens: Leafy green vegetables are not only rich in fiber but they are also rich in nitrates. Examples are kale, spinach, coriander, broccoli, cabbages, lettuce, mint, perilla, and arugula.

Carrots: This root vegetable is not only rich in vitamin A but is also high in nitrates.

Radishes: Radishes are another root vegetable that is a good source of nitrates for Nitric Oxide Synthesis.

Eggplants: This nightshade vegetable is an excellent source of nitrates. For a hundred grams of eggplant serving, you can get about 25-42 mg of nitrates.

Watermelon: Incorporating watermelon into your diet can help significantly in increasing the nitric oxide in your body.

Dark chocolate: Dark chocolate is also a good source of nitric oxide. It contains flavonoids, specifically epicatechins, which are known to boost the production of nitric oxide in the body.

Green tea: Green tea has been found to have a positive effect on nitric oxide levels. It contains a significant amount of flavonoids and antioxidants that are known to enhance the bioavailability of nitric oxide.

Berries: Berries, such as strawberries, raspberries, and blueberries, are a great source of dietary nitrate and antioxidants, which can help increase the production of nitric oxide in your body.

Incorporating nitric oxide-boosting foods into your diet

Here are some tips on how to incorporate these nitric oxide-boosting foods into your diet:

Start your day with a smoothie

Berries, spinach, and beetroots are all high in nitrates, which can boost nitric oxide levels in your body. Blend these ingredients together with a banana or Greek yogurt for a tasty, nutrient-dense breakfast.

Eat a variety of fruits and vegetables

Eating a variety of fruits and vegetables offers a lot of health benefits. Not only do they improve your skin health and promote gut health, but fruits and vegetables are often rich in nitrates. Always aim to add 2-3 cups of vegetables and 2.5-2 cups of fruits to your diet each day.

Include leafy greens in your meal

Incorporating leafy greens into each meal assures you you're boosting your Nitric Oxide production. Whether it's salad, smoothies, or stir-fry, always include in your 2-3 cups of daily vegetable intake a heap of leafy greens.

Add beets to your diet

As mentioned, beets are rich in nutrients and nitrates essential for Nitric Oxide production. There are a variety of ways to incorporate this delicious vegetable into your diet. You can try making chips out of it using your air fryer. Beet chips are the best alternative to processed and salted chips. It also makes a vibrant red juice or you could just boil or roast it.

Snack on nuts and seeds

Walnuts, pumpkin seeds, and sunflower seeds are rich in arginine, an amino acid that your body can convert into nitric oxide. These make for a healthy and satisfying snack.

Choose lean protein sources

Foods like poultry, fish, and lean cuts of meat are high in coenzyme Q10, which can help maintain nitric oxide levels. Include these in your meals regularly.

Spice it up with cayenne pepper

Cayenne pepper is rich in capsaicin, a compound that can stimulate nitric oxide production. Add it to your dishes for a spicy kick and health boost.

Drink pomegranate juice

Drinking pomegranate juice offers a lot of health benefits. This fruit is known to be an antioxidant and anti-inflammatory, promotes a healthy gut, and is rich in nitrate. Aside from making juice out of it, you could also add it to your salad.

Use garlic in cooking

Not only does garlic add aroma and flavor to your dishes, but it also has amino acids that are beneficial to your health. Garlic chips also make a delicious alternative to processed chips.

Snacks on citrus fruits

Citrus fruits like oranges and grapefruits make a delicious and healthy snack. Eat them guilt-free throughout the day to increase your Nitric Oxide.

Eat dark chocolate

Dark chocolate is not only delicious but also rich in flavonoids that can boost nitric oxide levels. Enjoy a small piece as a dessert or snack.

Incorporating Nitric Oxide-boosting foods into your diet is a convenient way to increase your NO synthesis.

Nitric Oxide Supplements: Pros and Cons

Nitric Oxide supplements have gained traction throughout the years in enhancing athletic performance, cardiovascular health, cognitive function, and immunity. But before you and your GP decide to opt for NO supplements, it is best that you both discuss its pros and cons.

Advantages of Nitric Oxide supplements

Here are some of the advantages that nitric oxide supplements could offer:

Targeted support

NO supplements can provide targeted and efficient support for specific health goals, such as improving athletic performance, endurance, and muscle recovery time, or reducing the risk of heart disease by improving cardiovascular health.

Convenience

Compared to diet and other lifestyle changes, taking nitric oxide supplements is convenient, especially for those individuals who have busy schedules or with dietary restrictions.

Efficiency

With the targeted support, NO supplements are more efficient in achieving your health goals compared to diet and lifestyle changes alone.

Variety

Nitric Oxide supplements come in various forms including, tablets, capsules, and powders, allowing individuals to choose what works best for them.

Potential risks and side effects of Nitric Oxide Supplements

While opting for Nitric Oxide supplements has advantages, it also comes with potential risks and side effects.

Low Blood Pressure

NO supplements may lower blood pressure, which can be dangerous for individuals with low blood pressure or those taking medication for high blood pressure.

Allergies

Nitric Oxide supplements may contain compounds that can cause an allergic reaction in some individuals. It is best that you discuss with your healthcare provider your history of allergies to identify what variant of NO supplement is best for you.

Interactions with medications

NO supplements may interact with certain medications, including blood thinners and erectile dysfunction medications. Always discuss with your healthcare provider the medications that you're currently taking.

Gastrointestinal issues

When taking Nitric Oxide supplements, watch out for any gastrointestinal issues such as nausea and diarrhea. Be sure to discuss any observed side effects with your GP.

Proper dosage and usage guidelines

Before taking any supplements, this must be done with guidance from your healthcare provider. Always follow the recommended dosage and usage guidelines on the label and the advice given by your doctor. Some healthcare professionals would also recommend cycling to maintain the supplement's efficacy and prevent your body from being accustomed to the medication.

Choosing a reputable brand

Your doctor may prescribe a generic brand of your Nitric Oxide supplement. Do your research if you want to go for branded ones. See if the NO supplement is from a reputable manufacturer, is certified by a third-party organization such as NSF International or USP, and contains high-quality ingredients.

In conclusion, while there are potential benefits to taking nitric oxide supplements, individuals should weigh these advantages against the potential risks and side effects, and choose a reputable brand while following proper dosage and usage guidelines. Consulting with a healthcare provider before starting to take NO supplements is highly recommended.

Who should not be taking Nitric Oxide Supplements?

While Nitric Oxide supplements are generally considered to be safe, several individuals should avoid taking these supplements. Nitric Oxide supplements may cause stomach discomfort, diarrhea, or allergies as mentioned above. It is best to consult your general practitioner if you're one of the following:

People with liver problems

The liver plays a crucial role in detoxifying the body, metabolizing drugs, and processing nutrients. Those individuals with underlying liver issues should steer clear from taking Nitric Oxide supplements. It is thought that Nitric Oxide supplements can negatively impact the liver especially if it's already compromised.

A compromised liver may inefficiently process substances such as NO supplements which can lead to the accumulation of unnecessary compounds that could exacerbate existing liver conditions. Therefore, it is best to talk to your doctor before taking any supplements if you have underlying liver issues.

People with low blood pressure or other heart problems

Nitric oxide plays a critical role in vascular health by helping to relax and widen blood vessels, thereby promoting better blood flow. While this is generally beneficial, it can cause problems for people with low blood pressure (hypotension) or certain heart conditions. Nitric oxide supplements can further lower blood pressure, leading to symptoms like dizziness, fainting, or even shock.

Similarly, for those with heart conditions, particularly those involving the heart valves or those with congestive heart failure, the additional dilation of blood vessels could put extra strain on the heart. Therefore, these individuals should avoid nitric oxide supplements unless under the supervision of a healthcare professional.

Individuals on medication for diabetes

As mentioned above, Nitric Oxide supplements can intervene with any current medications, especially for those who are taking medication for diabetes. Diabetes medications are for controlling blood sugar levels while Nitric Oxide's role is to regulate the blood flow. An enhanced blood flow could potentially decrease the cells' ability to absorb the medication or absorb the blood sugar as is supposed to be the function of diabetes medications. This could lead to an unpredictable fluctuation of sugar in the blood. If you're a diabetic and want to try Nitric Oxide supplements, please consult your doctor first.

Before undergoing surgery

Surgery puts the body under immense stress, requiring careful management of various physiological parameters, including blood pressure and clotting. Nitric oxide supplements, due to their blood pressure-lowering effects, could complicate surgical procedures and anesthesia management. Therefore, doctors typically recommend avoiding nitric oxide supplements in the weeks leading up to surgery. After surgery, once recovery is well underway and with the approval of a healthcare professional, these supplements can usually be safely reintroduced.

To cap it off, while Nitric Oxide supplements are considered safe, it is not suitable for everyone. It can cause side effects to individuals with underlying liver issues, low blood pressure, diabetes medication, and incoming surgery. It is important to speak with your doctor to discuss any underlying issues that may be triggered when taking Nitric Oxide supplements.

Nitric Oxide-Boosting Meal Recipes

The following pages contain some Nitric Oxide-boosting meal recipes that you can try. There are a variety of recipes to choose from, from smoothies to meals you can include in your diet. These are great options for you to kick-off your Nitric Oxide-rich diet.

Beet and Carrot Roast with Rosemary Garlic Butter

Ingredients:

- 2 medium beets
- 4 large carrots
- 2 tablespoons of rosemary garlic butter
- Salt and pepper to taste

Instructions:

1. Preheat your oven to 400 degrees Fahrenheit.
2. Peel and cut the beets and carrots into chunks.
3. Toss the vegetables in rosemary garlic butter, salt, and pepper.
4. Roast for 45 minutes or until the vegetables are tender.

Overnight Nitric Oxide Oats

Ingredients:

- 1 cup oats
- 2 cups almond milk
- 1 cup spinach
- 1 cup red spinach (aka. Amaranth)
- 1 cup arugula

Instructions:

1. Combine oats and almond milk in a bowl.
2. Cover and leave in the fridge overnight.
3. In the morning, top with spinach, red spinach, and arugula before eating.

Garlic and Leafy Greens Stir-fry

Ingredients:

- 2 cloves of garlic
- 2 cups of leafy greens, such as spinach, bok choy, etc.
- 1 tablespoon of olive oil
- Salt and pepper to taste

Instructions:

1. Heat olive oil in a pan.
2. Add garlic and sauté until fragrant.
3. Add leafy greens and stir-fry until wilted.
4. Season with salt and pepper.

Citrus Fruit Salad

Ingredients:

- 1 grapefruit
- 2 oranges
- 1 lime
- 1 lemon
- Honey to taste

Instructions:

1. Peel and slice all the fruits.
2. Combine in a bowl and drizzle with honey.

Watermelon and Pomegranate Smoothie

Ingredients:

- 2 cups watermelon cubes
- 1 cup pomegranate seeds
- 1 cup ice

Instructions:

1. Combine all ingredients in a blender.
2. Blend until smooth.
3. Serve immediately.

Beetroot and Orange Salad

Ingredients:

- 2 medium beetroot
- 2 oranges
- A handful of fresh mint leaves
- Olive oil and vinegar for dressing

Instructions:

1. Roast the beetroot in the oven until tender.
2. Peel and slice the oranges.
3. Once the beetroot has cooled, slice it and add to a bowl with the oranges and mint.
4. Drizzle with olive oil and vinegar before serving.

Spinach and Garlic Stuffed Chicken

Ingredients:

- 2 chicken breasts
- 2 cups of spinach
- 2 cloves of garlic
- Salt and pepper to taste

Instructions:

1. Preheat your oven to 375 degrees Fahrenheit.
2. Cut a slit in each chicken breast and stuff with spinach and garlic.
3. Season with salt and pepper.
4. Bake for 25-30 minutes or until the chicken is cooked through.

Dark Chocolate Avocado Mousse

Ingredients:

- 2 ripe avocados
- 1/2 cup unsweetened dark cocoa powder
- 1/2 cup honey or maple syrup
- 1 tsp vanilla extract

Instructions:

1. Combine all ingredients in a blender.
2. Blend until smooth.
3. Chill in the refrigerator before serving.

Pomegranate and Walnut Salad

Ingredients:

- 2 cups mixed salad greens
- 1 pomegranate
- 1/2 cup walnuts
- Olive oil and vinegar for dressing

Instructions:

1. Place the salad greens in a bowl.
2. Top with pomegranate seeds and walnuts.
3. Drizzle with olive oil and vinegar.

Watermelon, Mint, and Feta Salad

Ingredients:

- 2 cups diced watermelon
- A handful of fresh mint leaves
- 1/2 cup feta cheese
- Olive oil and vinegar for dressing

Instructions:

1. Combine the watermelon, mint, and feta in a bowl.
2. Drizzle with olive oil and vinegar before serving.

Spinach Berry Lemon Smoothie

Ingredients:

- 2 cups fresh spinach leaves, rinsed and roughly chopped
- 7–8 frozen strawberries
- 1 tbsp. chia seeds
- 1 tbsp. lemon juice
- 1 frozen banana, sliced
- 2–3 cups coconut water, chilled

Instructions:

1. Put the spinach leaves into the blender.
2. Add the banana, strawberries, lemon juice, chia seeds, and coconut water.
3. Blend well.
4. Serve and enjoy!

Pomegranate Refreshing Smoothie

Ingredients:

- 2 grapefruits
- 1/2 pomegranate
- 3 large collard leaves
- 1 cup coconut water

Instructions:

1. Put all ingredients in a blender.
2. Blend well.
3. Serve and enjoy.

Mediterranean Summer Salad

Ingredients:

- 3-4 cups leafy greens of your choice
- 6 tbsp. soft goat cheese
- fresh ground black pepper
- fresh cilantro, finely chopped
- 1 medium to large-sized red or golden beet

Avocado dressing:

- 1 small ripe avocado, halved and pit removed
- 1 tbsp. parsley, chopped
- 1 tbsp. cilantro, chopped
- 1 tbsp. lime juice
- 2 tbsp. rice vinegar
- 1/2 cup olive oil
- salt
- pepper

Lentil marinade:

- 1/4 cup French lentils
- 1/4 cup fennel, chopped,
- 1/2 cup zucchini, chopped
- 1-2 pcs. shallots, chopped
- 2 tbsp. dill
- hing
- salt

- pepper
- 1 cup water
- 1 tbsp. rice vinegar
- 2 tsp. olive oil
- sunflower oil

Couscous:

- 1/2 cup Israeli or pearl couscous
- 2 tbsp. chopped parsley
- 3/4 cup water or broth
- 2 tsp. sunflower oil
- 1/2 tsp. salt
- 1/4 tsp. pepper
- 1/2 lemon, juice only

Instructions:

For the lentil marinade:

1. In a pot, simmer the following for about 20 minutes: water, lentils, and a pinch of hing.
2. In a bowl, mix fennel, dill, rice vinegar, olive oil, and a dash of salt and pepper.
3. In a saucepan, saute lightly the following: sunflower oil, zucchini, shallots, and rice vinegar.
4. Let everything cool down before mixing it together.
5. Place the marinade in the refrigerator overnight or for at least 4 hours.

For the couscous:

1. Saute couscous in sunflower oil for about 2-3 minutes.
2. Pour water or broth and bring to a boil.
3. Lower the heat and allow to simmer for about 10-15 minutes.
4. Add in parsley and lemon juice, then season with salt and pepper.
5. This may be served warm or prepared earlier and refrigerated to be served later.

For the beet:

1. Cut the beet into quarters. Peel off the outer layer.
2. In a steamer, add water until it's about an inch high.
3. Place the beets in the steamer and steam until done, or about 20 minutes.
4. After cooling down, chop the beets into 1/2-inch sizes.
5. Store in the refrigerator before serving.

For the avocado dressing:

1. Scoop out avocado flesh using a teaspoon.
2. Put avocado flesh in a food processor or blender, followed by the rest of the ingredients.
3. Blend everything until it is smooth and mixed well.
4. Season with salt and pepper before serving.

To make the salad:

1. On a serving bowl or plate, toss together the greens and the dressing.
2. Layer on top the prepared lentil marinade, couscous, and beets.
3. Add the goat cheese all around the platter, then finish off with a dash of pepper and cilantro before serving.

Energy Boost Smoothie

Ingredients:

- 1 large rib celery
- 1 tablespoon parsley
- 3/4 cup water
- 1/2 cup chopped cooked beets
- 1 small orange, segmented
- 3/4 cup chopped carrot

Instructions:

1. Using a blender, mix the water, parsley, and celery. Increase speed until all solid particles are gone.
2. Add the rest of the ingredients. Resume blending until reaching the maximum speed.
3. Maintain the maximum speed for 30 seconds before serving.
4. Serve chilled.

Anti-Diabetic Smoothie

Ingredients:

- 2 cups spinach
- 2 large kale leaves
- 3/4 cup water
- 1 large frozen banana
- 1/2 cup frozen mango
- 1/2 cup frozen peach
- 1 tbsp. ground flaxseeds
- 1 tbsp. almond butter or peanut butter

Instructions:

1. Using a blender, mix the water, spinach, and kale. Increase speed until all solid particles are gone.
2. Add the rest of the ingredients. Resume blending until reaching the maximum speed.
3. Maintain the maximum speed for 30 seconds before serving.
4. Serve chilled.

Detox Juice

Ingredients:

- 1 beet, scrubbed
- 1 apple
- 1 lemon, peeled
- 1 cucumber, peeled
- one handful of dandelion greens, washed

Instruction:

Juice everything and stir well.

Spinach and Kale Blend

Ingredients:

- 1 cup spinach
- 1 cup chopped kale
- 3/4 cup water
- 1/2 cup chopped cucumber
- 1 green apple
- 1 cup chopped papaya
- 1 tbsp. ground flaxseed

Instructions:

1. Using a blender, mix water, spinach, and kale. Increase speed until all solid particles are gone.
2. Add the rest of the ingredients. Resume blending until reaching the maximum speed.
3. Maintain the maximum speed for 30 seconds before serving.
4. Serve chilled.

Strawberries and Elderberry Puree

Ingredients:

- 1 cup frozen strawberries, quartered
- 4 cups filtered water
- 1/4 cup salad-grade elderberry flowers, rinsed well and drained

Instructions:

1. Place all ingredients into a large pitcher. Mix while gently bruising berries.
2. Set aside for at least an hour in the fridge.
3. Strain out flowers. Pour drink. Consume liquid and berries.
4. Serve and enjoy.

Low FODMAP Blueberry Smoothie

Ingredients:

- 1 cup frozen blueberries
- 1 tbsp. almond butter
- 1/2 cup almond milk

Instructions:

1. Throw all the ingredients into a blender.
2. Blend on high until creamy and smooth.
3. Serve immediately. Top with blueberries if you want.

Blueberry Flax Smoothie

Ingredients:

- 1 cup blueberries, frozen
- 1 tbsp. flaxseed, ground
- a handful of spinach leaves
- 1/4 cup full-fat Greek yogurt
- 1 cup coconut milk or any kind of milk

Instruction:

Place all ingredients in a blender or magic bullet. Mix until smooth.

Conclusion

And there you have it! You have reached the culmination of this guide. Congratulations on making it this far in your journey towards healthy well-being with Nitric Oxide.

This signaling molecule offers a wide range of benefits to your health such as enhanced exercise performance, improved cardiovascular health, better cognitive function, and strong immunity. In this sense, Nitric Oxide is worth exploring, especially for athletes, individuals with hypertension, and anyone who wants to improve their overall health.

Now that you have done your research, you're equipped with knowledge on how to boost your body's NO levels. Whether you opt for diet and lifestyle changes, or Nitric Oxide supplements, be sure to evaluate and identify your health goals. A healthcare professional's guidance is also important throughout this process. While taking the NO supplements is convenient and could be efficient, it is best to weigh the pros and cons that come with it.

Incorporating Nitric Oxide-boosting foods into your diet is a natural way of increasing your NO levels while acquiring the essential nutrients that are beneficial to your overall well-being. Exercise, adequate hydration, getting enough sunlight, sufficient sleep, and quitting smoke are lifestyle changes that you could also do right now aside from a healthy diet to promote healthy levels of Nitric Oxide in your body.

Your health goals are your motivation in this journey and we hope that this guide is instrumental to achieving it.

FAQ

What is Nitric Oxide?

Nitric Oxide is a simple molecule that is responsible for regulating the blood flow throughout your body. It is one of those signaling molecules that promotes vasodilation.

What are the benefits of Nitric Oxide?

Nitric Oxide is beneficial in cardiovascular health, cognitive function, immunity, erectile function, and enhanced physiological activities.

How can I increase the Nitric Oxide levels in my body?

You can increase your Nitric Oxide levels by incorporating Nitrate-rich foods into your diet, exercising, getting enough sleep, adequate hydration, enough sunlight exposure, and quitting smoke. You can also opt for NO supplements with your healthcare provider's guidance.

Can you give me examples of nitrate-rich foods?

Some of the nitrate-rich foods are green leafy vegetables, citrus fruits, pomegranate, garlic, carrots, radishes, and beets.

Are there side effects in taking NO supplements?

While taking NO supplements has advantages such as convenience and efficiency, it also comes with potential risks and side effects including low blood pressure, gastrointestinal issues, allergies, and interactions with other medications. It is best that you weigh these pros and cons with your doctor.

Can I take NO supplements while taking medications for my diabetes?

Nitric Oxide supplements enhance the blood flow which may be able to reduce the efficacy of your diabetes medication. It is best to speak and discuss this with your doctor.

References and Helpful Links

Chen, K., Pittman, R. N., & Popel, A. S. (2008). Nitric oxide in the vasculature: Where does it come from and where does it go? A quantitative perspective. Antioxidants & Redox Signaling, 10(7), 1185–1198. https://doi.org/10.1089/ars.2007.1959

Hudgens, S. (2023). What is nitric oxide? Health. https://www.health.com/nitric-oxide-7557367

Bcps, R. P. P. B. B. (2023). Nitric Oxide: Everything you need to know. Verywell Health. https://www.verywellhealth.com/nitric-oxide-everything-you-need-to-know-7499807

Umipig, K. (2023). Top 10 foods to boost your nitric oxide levels. Longevity.Technology Lifestyle | Health, Fitness & Technology. https://longevity.technology/lifestyle/top-10-foods-to-boost-your-nitric-oxide-levels/

Zucker, J. (2023). The best nitric oxide foods to increase blood flow and boost performance. BarBend. https://barbend.com/best-nitric-oxide-foods/

Crna, R. N. M. (2023, April 14). What to know about nitric oxide supplements. https://www.medicalnewstoday.com/articles/326381

Van De Walle Ms Rd, G. (2023, February 28). 5 Ways nitric oxide supplements Boost your health and performance. Healthline. https://www.healthline.com/nutrition/nitric-oxide-supplements

www.ingramcontent.com/pod-product-compliance
Lightning Source LLC
LaVergne TN
LVHW012034060526
838201LV00061B/4611